THURSTAN DAVIES

The Carnivore Diet – A Comprehensive Guide

MEDICAL DISCLAIMER

The information provided in this book is for educational and informational purposes only and is not intended as medical advice. The Carnivore Diet, like any significant dietary change, may not be suitable for everyone, and individual results may vary. The author and publisher of this book are not medical professionals, and the content herein should not be construed as medical, health, or nutritional advice.

Before making any changes to your diet, lifestyle, or exercise routine, it is essential to consult with a qualified healthcare provider. This is particularly important if you have any existing health conditions, are taking medications, or have specific dietary requirements. A medical professional can provide personalized advice and guidance based on your individual health needs and medical history.

The Carnivore Diet may carry risks, including but not limited to potential nutrient deficiencies and other health concerns. It is crucial to approach any dietary change with caution and to monitor your health regularly. If you experience any adverse effects or have concerns about your health while following the Carnivore Diet, seek medical attention promptly.

The author and publisher disclaim any liability or loss in connection with the information provided in this book. The reader assumes full responsibility for any decisions or actions taken based on the content of this book. Always prioritize your health and well-being and seek professional medical advice as needed.

First edition

This book was professionally typeset on Reedsy.
Find out more at reedsy.com

To Alla,

This book is a testament to your belief in me. It stands as a symbol of our shared dreams and the incredible life we are building together. Thank you for being my muse, my confidante, and my greatest love. You are my heart, my inspiration, and the reason I strive for greatness.

With all the love and gratitude my heart can hold, I dedicate this book to you, my everything.

Forever yours,

Thurstan Davies
May 2024

Contents

INTRODUCTION

In a world where dietary advice is as varied as it is abundant, there exists a unique dietary paradigm that both challenges conventional wisdom and invites us to reconsider our relationship with food. This book, "The Carnivore Diet: A Comprehensive Guide" is an exploration of this audacious approach to nutrition, designed to inform, inspire, and empower readers to make informed decisions about their health and lifestyle.

The Call to Exploration

Imagine a world where every meal is a celebration of simplicity, where the focus is on nutrient-dense, unprocessed food that our ancestors might have recognized. The Carnivore Diet proposes such a world, one where animal-based foods are not only the foundation of our sustenance but also the key to unlocking optimal health. This book has been written to guide you through this dietary landscape, providing you with the knowledge, tools, and confidence to explore this unconventional yet profoundly impactful way of eating.

Why This Book?

In recent years, the Carnivore Diet has surged in popularity, capturing the interest of health enthusiasts, biohackers, and those seeking solutions to chronic health issues. Despite its growing following, comprehensive resources that delve deeply into the diet's history, science, and practical application are still scarce. This book aims to fill that gap, offering a detailed and nuanced exploration of the Carnivore Diet.

From the historical roots of our meat-eating ancestors to the latest scientific research, this guide covers all aspects of the Carnivore Diet. Each chapter is meticulously crafted to provide a blend of factual information, expert opinions, and real-life anecdotes, ensuring that you are well-equipped to understand and potentially embrace this lifestyle.

What You Will Discover

Our journey begins with a deep dive into the history and evolution of the Carnivore Diet. We will trace the dietary patterns of early humans and explore how traditional societies thrived on predominantly meat-based diets. This historical context sets the stage for understanding the diet's modern resurgence and the key figures who have brought it into the limelight.

Next, we will delve into the science behind the Carnivore Diet. By examining the physiological and biochemical impacts of an all-meat diet, we will uncover the mechanisms through which it can potentially promote health and well-being. This chapter will be grounded in contemporary research and expert insights, providing a solid scientific foundation for the diet's principles.

The health benefits of the Carnivore Diet will be explored in detail, highlighting its potential to improve various aspects of health, from metabolic function to mental clarity. We will also address common health concerns and myths, presenting a balanced view of the diet's potential advantages.

No discussion of the Carnivore Diet would be complete without addressing its potential risks and criticisms. This chapter will provide a critical analysis of the diet's limitations and the concerns raised by health professionals and sceptics. By acknowledging these critiques, we aim to present a well-rounded perspective that empowers you to make informed decisions.

For those ready to embark on their Carnivore journey, the practical aspects of getting started will be covered in detail. From transitioning tips to essential kitchen staples, this chapter will provide a step-by-step guide to adopting the Carnivore Diet with confidence and ease.

To keep your culinary experience both delightful and varied, we have included a chapter dedicated to meal plans and recipes. Here, you will find creative and delicious ways to prepare and enjoy meat-based meals, ensuring that your diet remains enjoyable and sustainable.

Recognizing the importance of a holistic approach to health, we will also explore how to integrate exercise with the Carnivore Diet. This chapter will offer insights into optimizing physical performance and recovery, tailored specifically to those following an all-meat diet.

We will then turn our focus to specific populations, such as athletes, older adults, and individuals with chronic illnesses, discussing how the Carnivore Diet can be adapted to meet their unique needs. This chapter will provide valuable insights for anyone considering the diet, regardless of their life stage or health status.

The social and psychological aspects of the Carnivore Diet will also be addressed, as we understand that dietary changes can impact more than just physical health. We will explore how to navigate social situations, manage cravings, and maintain a positive relationship with food while adhering to the Carnivore Diet.

Looking ahead, we will speculate on the future of the Carnivore Diet. With advancements in nutritional science and a growing community of advocates, we will discuss how the diet might evolve and its potential role in the broader context of health and wellness trends.

In our bonus chapter, we will provide practical tips for sustaining the Carnivore

Diet in the long term. This chapter will offer strategies for overcoming challenges, staying motivated, and ensuring nutritional adequacy over time.

Transition to Chapter 1: The History and Evolution of the Carnivore Diet

As we embark on this journey together, let us first turn our attention to the past. Understanding the historical context of the Carnivore Diet not only grounds us in its origins but also provides valuable insights into its potential benefits. In the next chapter, we will explore the dietary practices of early humans and traditional societies, and how their meat-based diets laid the foundation for the modern Carnivore movement. Join us as we travel back in time to uncover the roots of this ancient and enduring dietary approach.

ONE | The History and Evolution of the Carnivore Diet

The Dawn of Human Diets

To truly grasp the essence of the Carnivore Diet, we must embark on a journey back to the origins of humanity itself. Picture early humans—nomadic hunter-gatherers—traversing the vast savannas and dense forests of prehistoric Earth. These early ancestors, driven by survival instincts and equipped with rudimentary tools, relied heavily on meat for sustenance. Their dietary choices were dictated not by modern nutritional guidelines but by the harsh realities of their environment.

Tracing the Roots: Early Human Diets

Anthropological evidence suggests that early humans, such as Homo habilis and Homo erectus, were predominantly meat-eaters. The development of tools and the ability to hunt large game marked a significant shift in our evolutionary journey. The consumption of nutrient-dense animal flesh provided the essential proteins and fats required for the growth of our brains and bodies. This dietary adaptation is believed to have given Homo sapiens a substantial evolutionary advantage.

Fossil records and archaeological findings indicate that meat constituted a significant portion of the diet of these early humans. Cut marks on animal bones and the presence of hunting tools in ancient sites reveal a clear preference for meat consumption. This reliance on meat was not merely a dietary choice but a necessity for survival in a world where plant-based foods were often scarce or seasonal.

Traditional Societies and Meat-Based Diets

Fast forward to more recent history, and we find numerous traditional societies that thrived on predominantly meat-based diets. These cultures offer invaluable insights into the sustainability and health impacts of such a dietary approach.

The Inuit: Masters of the Arctic

The Inuit, indigenous to the Arctic regions of Greenland, Canada, and Alaska, have long been celebrated for their ability to thrive in one of the harshest environments on Earth. With limited access to plant-based foods, the Inuit diet historically consisted almost entirely of animal products, including fish, seals, whales, and caribou.

The Inuit's remarkable health and endurance were attributed to their high-fat, low-carbohydrate diet. Despite consuming large amounts of animal fat, traditional Inuit populations exhibited low rates of heart disease and maintained robust physical health. This paradox challenges conventional dietary wisdom and highlights the potential benefits of a meat-based diet.

The Maasai: Warriors of East Africa

In the grasslands of East Africa, the Maasai people have sustained themselves on a diet rich in animal products for centuries. Renowned for their tall stature and physical prowess, the Maasai primarily consume meat, milk, and blood from their cattle.

The Maasai's diet is high in saturated fat, yet studies have shown that they have low incidences of cardiovascular disease. This apparent contradiction has sparked interest and debate among researchers, prompting a re-evaluation of the relationship between dietary fats and heart health.

The Sami: Reindeer Herders of Scandinavia

The Sami people, indigenous to the Arctic and sub-Arctic regions of Scandinavia, have traditionally relied on reindeer for their sustenance. The Sami diet includes reindeer meat, fish, and other animal products, providing a rich source of protein and fat essential for survival in cold climates.

The Sami's reliance on animal-based foods underscores the adaptability of human diets to different environmental conditions. Their dietary practices offer a glimpse into how traditional meat-based diets can support health and vitality in diverse settings.

The Modern Resurgence of the Carnivore Diet

While traditional societies provide historical context, the modern resurgence of the Carnivore Diet is a relatively recent phenomenon. Over the past few decades, interest in low-carbohydrate and ketogenic diets has paved the way for the revival of the Carnivore Diet. This contemporary movement is driven by a combination of anecdotal success stories, scientific inquiry, and the influence of key figures who have championed the diet.

Key Figures in the Carnivore Movement

Several individuals have played pivotal roles in popularizing the Carnivore Diet, bringing it from the fringes of dietary experimentation to the mainstream.

Dr Shawn Baker: A Catalyst for Change

Dr Shawn Baker, an orthopaedic surgeon and former athlete, is perhaps the most well-known advocate of the Carnivore Diet. His personal journey of transforming his health and fitness through an all-meat diet has inspired thousands to explore this unconventional approach.

Baker's book, "The Carnivore Diet," and his active presence on social media have provided a platform for sharing the benefits of the diet, backed by both scientific insights and personal anecdotes. His emphasis on the simplicity and effectiveness of a meat-based diet resonates with many seeking to improve their health.

Mikhaila Peterson: A Personal Transformation

Mikhaila Peterson, the daughter of psychologist Jordan Peterson, has also been a prominent voice in the Carnivore community. Battling severe autoimmune and mental health issues, Mikhaila turned to a strict Carnivore Diet and experienced dramatic improvements in her health.

Her story, widely shared through her blog and interviews, has highlighted the potential of the Carnivore Diet to address chronic health conditions. Mikhaila's journey underscores the diet's transformative power and its potential to offer hope to those struggling with similar issues.

Dr Paul Saladino: The Carnivore MD

Dr Paul Saladino, a physician specializing in integrative medicine, has become a leading authority on the Carnivore Diet. Through his book "The Carnivore Code" and his podcast, Saladino delves into the science behind the diet, advocating for its benefits based on evolutionary principles and modern research.

Saladino's work has helped bridge the gap between anecdotal evidence and scientific validation, providing a more comprehensive understanding of how and why the Carnivore Diet can be beneficial.

The Role of Social Media and Online Communities

The rise of social media and online communities has been instrumental in spreading the message of the Carnivore Diet. Platforms like Instagram, YouTube, and Facebook have allowed individuals to share their experiences, successes, and challenges, fostering a supportive and informative network for those interested in the diet.

Challenges and Criticisms

Despite its growing popularity, the Carnivore Diet is not without its detractors. Critics argue that the diet is too restrictive and lacks essential nutrients found in plant-based foods. Concerns about long-term health effects, sustainability, and ethical considerations also fuel the debate.

However, proponents counter these criticisms by pointing to historical precedents, scientific studies, and personal success stories that highlight the diet's potential benefits. The ongoing discourse underscores the need for more research and open-minded exploration of different dietary approaches.

Conclusion: A Diet Rooted in History and Revitalized by Modern Science

The history and evolution of the Carnivore Diet provide a fascinating backdrop for understanding its contemporary resurgence. From the diets of our early ancestors to the practices of traditional societies, the reliance on meat as a primary food source has deep roots. The modern revival, championed by key figures and amplified by social media, offers a compelling alternative to conventional dietary wisdom.

As we move forward, it is essential to balance historical insights with modern scientific inquiry, embracing a holistic and nuanced view of the Carnivore Diet. In the next chapter, we will delve deeper into the scientific foundations of the diet, exploring how it impacts our bodies and health. Join us as we uncover the mechanisms that make the Carnivore Diet a subject of growing interest and debate in the world of nutrition.

TWO | The Science Behind the Carnivore Diet

The Biological Symphony of the Carnivore Diet

Understanding the biological mechanisms behind the Carnivore Diet is not only fascinating but also crucial for appreciating its potential benefits and risks. This chapter will unravel the science that underpins this unique dietary approach, exploring macronutrients, metabolic processes, and how the body adapts to an all-meat diet. We will also compare the Carnivore Diet with other popular low-carb diets such as Keto and Paleo, highlighting what sets this diet apart.

Macronutrients: The Building Blocks of the Carnivore Diet

At the heart of the Carnivore Diet lies a focus on two primary macronutrients: proteins and fats. Carbohydrates, a staple in many modern diets, are virtually non-existent in this dietary plan. To understand how the Carnivore Diet functions, we must first dissect these macronutrients and their roles in the body.

Proteins: The Body's Building Blocks

Proteins are essential for the growth, repair, and maintenance of body tissues. They are composed of amino acids, which are often referred to as the building blocks of life. Animal-based foods provide complete proteins, meaning they contain all the essential amino acids that the human body cannot synthesize on its own.

In the Carnivore Diet, protein sources such as beef, pork, poultry, and fish play a crucial role. These proteins support muscle growth, immune function, and the production of enzymes and hormones. Additionally, proteins have a high thermic effect, meaning the body burns more calories digesting protein compared to fats or carbohydrates, which can aid in weight management.

Fats: The Preferred Fuel

Fats, particularly saturated and monounsaturated fats found in animal products, are the primary energy source in the Carnivore Diet. These fats are vital for cell membrane integrity, hormone production, and the absorption of fat-soluble vitamins (A, D, E, and K).

Animal fats, such as those found in beef, pork, and fatty fish, provide a dense source of energy. When carbohydrates are restricted, the body shifts to burning fat for fuel, a process known as ketosis. This metabolic state not only supports energy levels but also has been linked to various health benefits, including improved mental clarity and reduced inflammation.

Carbohydrates: The Missing Macronutrient

In stark contrast to the standard Western diet, the Carnivore Diet eliminates carbohydrates almost entirely. This absence forces the body to adapt metabolically, shifting from glucose (derived from carbohydrates) to ketones (produced from fats) as its primary energy source.

Metabolic State of Ketosis

Ketosis is a metabolic state in which the liver converts fatty acids into ketones, which then serve as an alternative energy source for the body, particularly the brain. This state is achieved through significant carbohydrate restriction, which depletes glycogen stores in the liver and muscles.

The Benefits of Ketosis

The state of ketosis offers several benefits that align with the principles of the Carnivore Diet:

Enhanced Fat Burning: With carbohydrates restricted, the body becomes highly efficient at burning fat for fuel. This can lead to significant weight loss and improved body composition.

Stable Blood Sugar Levels: Ketosis helps maintain stable blood sugar levels, reducing insulin spikes and crashes associated with carbohydrate consumption. This can be particularly beneficial for individuals with insulin resistance or type 2 diabetes.

Improved Mental Clarity: Ketones are a more efficient fuel for the brain compared to glucose. Many individuals on the Carnivore Diet report enhanced mental clarity, focus, and cognitive function.

Reduced Inflammation: Ketosis has been shown to reduce markers of inflammation in the body. This can lead to improvements in conditions such as arthritis, autoimmune diseases, and other inflammatory disorders.

Comparing the Carnivore Diet with Keto and Paleo

While the Carnivore Diet shares similarities with other low-carb diets such as Keto and Paleo, it also has distinct differences that set it apart.

The Ketogenic Diet

The Ketogenic (Keto) Diet is characterized by a high-fat, moderate-protein, and very low-carbohydrate intake. The goal of the Keto Diet is to induce and maintain a state of ketosis. While both the Keto and Carnivore diets aim to achieve ketosis, there are key differences:

Macronutrient Ratios: The Keto Diet typically includes a higher proportion of fats to proteins, whereas the Carnivore Diet does not strictly regulate these ratios, allowing for more flexibility in protein intake.

Food Variety: The Keto Diet allows for a variety of low-carb vegetables, nuts, seeds, and dairy products. In contrast, the Carnivore Diet is strictly limited to animal-based foods, excluding all plant-based foods.

The Paleo Diet

The Paleo Diet, inspired by the dietary patterns of our Palaeolithic ancestors, emphasizes whole, unprocessed foods. It includes lean meats, fish, fruits, vegetables, nuts, and seeds while excluding processed foods, grains, legumes, and dairy.

Inclusion of Plant Foods: Unlike the Carnivore Diet, the Paleo Diet includes a wide variety of plant-based foods. This allows for a more balanced intake of nutrients, including fibre and phytonutrients.

Focus on Ancestral Eating: While both diets draw inspiration from ancestral eating patterns, the Paleo Diet aims to mimic the presumed diet of early humans more closely, incorporating a mix of animal and plant foods.

Unique Aspects of the Carnivore Diet

What sets the Carnivore Diet apart from Keto and Paleo is its extreme simplicity and exclusivity of animal-based foods. This singular focus has several implications:

Nutrient Density: *Animal-based foods are nutrient-dense, providing essential vitamins and minerals in highly bioavailable forms. For example, organ meats like liver are rich in vitamin A, iron, and B vitamins.*

Simplicity: *The Carnivore Diet eliminates the need for counting macros, tracking calories, or planning complex meals. This simplicity can be appealing to those who find traditional dieting methods cumbersome.*

Adaptation and Satiety: *Many adherents of the Carnivore Diet report a profound sense of satiety and reduced cravings. This could be attributed to the high protein and fat content of the diet, which promotes fullness and reduces the likelihood of overeating.*

Biochemical Adaptations

When transitioning to the Carnivore Diet, the body undergoes several biochemical adaptations. These changes are crucial for understanding how the diet affects overall health and performance.

Gluconeogenesis: *In the absence of dietary carbohydrates, the liver produces glucose from non-carbohydrate sources, such as amino acids. This process, known as gluconeogenesis, ensures that the body maintains adequate glucose levels for critical functions.*

Hormonal Adjustments: *The Carnivore Diet influences various hormones, including insulin, glucagon, and leptin. These hormonal changes contribute to improved insulin sensitivity, stable blood sugar levels, and enhanced satiety signals.*

Microbiome Shifts: *The gut microbiome adapts to the Carnivore Diet,* *shifting towards bacteria that thrive on animal-based foods. While this shift raises questions about long-term gut health, many individuals report improvements in digestive symptoms.*

Expert Opinions

The scientific community is divided on the Carnivore Diet. Some experts praise its potential benefits, particularly for metabolic health and weight management, while others caution against its restrictive nature and potential nutrient deficiencies.

Proponents' Views

Proponents argue that the Carnivore Diet aligns with our evolutionary history and offers a straightforward solution to modern health issues. They highlight its effectiveness in managing autoimmune diseases, improving mental health, and promoting sustainable weight loss.

Sceptics' Concerns

Sceptics, on the other hand, raise concerns about the lack of dietary fibre, potential vitamin and mineral deficiencies, and the unknown long-term health effects. They advocate for a more balanced approach that includes a variety of whole foods.

Conclusion: Embracing the Science

The science behind the Carnivore Diet is both intriguing and complex. By focusing on nutrient-dense animal-based foods and inducing a state of ketosis, this diet offers a unique approach to health and nutrition. However, it also challenges conventional dietary norms and requires careful consideration of its potential risks and benefits.

In the next chapter, we will explore the specific health benefits of the Carnivore Diet, supported by scientific studies and real-life testimonials. Join us as we delve into how this diet can improve metabolic health, mental clarity, and overall well-being, providing you with a deeper understanding of its transformative potential.

THREE | Health Benefits of the Carnivore Diet

The Potential Health Benefits of Embracing Carnivory

In a world overflowing with dietary options, the Carnivore Diet stands out as a bold, radical approach. By focusing exclusively on animal-based foods, proponents claim numerous health benefits, from weight loss to mental clarity and the management of chronic illnesses. This chapter delves into these potential benefits, supported by scientific evidence and real-life testimonials, to provide a comprehensive understanding of what the Carnivore Diet can offer.

Shedding Pounds: The Promise of Weight Loss

One of the most compelling reasons people turn to the Carnivore Diet is its potential for significant weight loss. The mechanics of this diet, high in protein and fat but devoid of carbohydrates, set the stage for effective weight management.

The Role of Ketosis

The Carnivore Diet induces a metabolic state known as ketosis. Without carbohydrates, the body begins to burn fat for fuel, producing ketones. This shift can lead to rapid and sustained weight loss as the body becomes efficient at utilizing stored fat.

Satiety and Reduced Cravings

High protein intake plays a crucial role in satiety. Proteins trigger the release of satiety hormones such as peptide YY and GLP-1, which signal the brain to stop eating. Additionally, the absence of carbohydrates prevents blood sugar spikes and crashes, reducing hunger and cravings.

Anecdotal Evidence: Transformative Weight Loss Stories

Countless individuals have shared their transformative weight loss journeys on the Carnivore Diet. For instance, Joe, a 42-year-old from Texas, struggled with obesity for years. After adopting the Carnivore Diet, he lost over 80 pounds in just 12 months. His story is echoed by many who find that the simplicity and effectiveness of the diet help them achieve and maintain a healthy weight.

Mental Clarity and Cognitive Function

Beyond physical benefits, the Carnivore Diet is reputed to enhance mental clarity and cognitive function. This aspect is particularly appealing to those seeking improved focus, memory, and overall brain health.

Ketones as Brain Fuel

Ketones, produced during ketosis, are a more efficient and stable source of energy for the brain than glucose. Studies have shown that ketones can enhance cognitive function and protect against neurodegenerative diseases. The brain's preference for ketones over glucose may explain the reported improvements in mental clarity and focus.

Reduced Brain Fog and Enhanced Mood

Many adherents of the Carnivore Diet report a significant reduction in brain fog. This could be attributed to the stabilization of blood sugar levels and the elimination of inflammatory foods. Additionally, the diet's high intake of omega-3 fatty acids from fish and grass-fed meats supports brain health and mood regulation.

Testimonial: A Clearer Mind

Mikhaila Peterson, who popularized the diet through her blog and interviews, has shared how the Carnivore Diet dramatically improved her mental health. Struggling with severe depression and brain fog, she experienced a newfound clarity and stability in her mood after transitioning to an all-meat diet. Her story is a testament to the potential cognitive benefits of the Carnivore Diet.

Managing Chronic Illnesses: Autoimmune Diseases and Diabetes

The Carnivore Diet's impact on chronic illnesses is a burgeoning field of interest. While more research is needed, early evidence and numerous testimonials suggest that this diet can offer significant relief for conditions such as autoimmune diseases and diabetes.

Autoimmune Diseases

Autoimmune diseases occur when the body's immune system mistakenly attacks its tissues. Diet plays a critical role in managing these conditions, as certain foods can trigger inflammatory responses.

Elimination of Inflammatory Foods

The Carnivore Diet eliminates common inflammatory foods, such as grains, dairy, and processed foods. By doing so, it may reduce the inflammatory burden on the body, allowing the immune system to reset and function correctly.

Real-Life Testimonial: Mikhaila Peterson

Mikhaila Peterson's journey with the Carnivore Diet began as a quest to manage her autoimmune conditions. Plagued by juvenile rheumatoid arthritis and chronic fatigue, she turned to an all-meat diet. The results were profound—her symptoms dramatically reduced, and she was able to taper off her medications. Her experience highlights the potential of the Carnivore Diet to manage and even reverse autoimmune conditions.

Diabetes Management

The Carnivore Diet's ability to stabilize blood sugar levels makes it a promising option for managing diabetes, particularly type 2 diabetes.

Stabilizing Blood Sugar

By eliminating carbohydrates, the primary driver of blood sugar spikes, the Carnivore Diet helps maintain stable blood sugar levels. This stabilization reduces the need for insulin, allowing individuals with type 2 diabetes to better manage their condition.

Improved Insulin Sensitivity

High protein and fat intake improve insulin sensitivity, further aiding in the management of diabetes. Improved insulin sensitivity means the body can utilize insulin more effectively, reducing the risk of insulin resistance.

Testimonial: Reversing Diabetes

John, a 55-year-old from California, was diagnosed with type 2 diabetes a decade ago. Despite following conventional dietary advice, his condition worsened. After switching to the Carnivore Diet, John experienced a remarkable improvement—his blood sugar levels normalized, and he was able to reduce his insulin dosage significantly. His story mirrors that of many who have found hope in the Carnivore Diet for managing diabetes.

Cardiovascular Health: A Counter-intuitive Benefit

While the Carnivore Diet's high intake of saturated fats has raised concerns, emerging evidence suggests that it may benefit cardiovascular health in unexpected ways.

Improved Cholesterol Profiles

Contrary to conventional wisdom, many individuals on the Carnivore Diet report improved cholesterol profiles. This includes increased HDL (good cholesterol) and decreased triglycerides, both of which are associated with a lower risk of heart disease.

Reduced Inflammation

Chronic inflammation is a known risk factor for cardiovascular disease. By reducing inflammatory markers, the Carnivore Diet may lower the risk of heart disease. Additionally, the elimination of processed foods and sugars contributes to this anti-inflammatory effect.

Case Study: Cardiovascular Health Improvements

A case study involving a 47-year-old man with a history of high cholesterol and hypertension showed remarkable improvements after six months on the Carnivore Diet. His LDL (bad cholesterol) levels decreased, HDL levels increased, and his blood pressure normalized. This case underscores the potential cardiovascular benefits of the Carnivore Diet, though more research is needed to generalize these findings.

Digestive Health: A Surprising Turnaround

The Carnivore Diet's impact on digestive health is another area where it has garnered positive testimonials. Many individuals report relief from chronic digestive issues such as irritable bowel syndrome (IBS) and bloating.

Simplified Digestion

Animal-based foods are easier for the body to digest and absorb. The simplicity of the Carnivore Diet reduces the digestive workload, potentially alleviating symptoms of digestive disorders.

Gut Health and Microbiome

While the long-term effects on the gut microbiome are still being studied, many report improved digestive health. The diet's high protein and fat content support the growth of beneficial gut bacteria, though it's crucial to monitor for any negative changes over time.

Testimonial: Digestive Relief

Emma, a 30-year-old from New York, struggled with IBS for years. After adopting the Carnivore Diet, she experienced significant relief from her symptoms. Her bloating subsided, and her bowel movements normalized. Emma's story is one of many that highlight the diet's potential to improve digestive health.

Conclusion: A Promising Yet Unconventional Approach

The health benefits of the Carnivore Diet are diverse and compelling. From weight loss and mental clarity to the management of chronic illnesses, this diet offers a unique approach to health and well-being. Supported by both scientific evidence and real-life testimonials, the Carnivore Diet presents itself as a promising, though unconventional, dietary option.

As we continue our exploration, the next chapter will address potential risks and criticisms of the Carnivore Diet. Understanding these challenges is crucial for making an informed decision about whether this diet is right for you. Join us as we delve into the potential downsides and how to navigate them effectively.

FOUR | Potential Risks and Criticisms

A Balanced View: Unveiling the Potential Risks of the Carnivore Diet

As alluring as the Carnivore Diet may seem, with its promises of weight loss, mental clarity, and relief from chronic ailments, it is not without its critics. Every dietary approach carries inherent risks and potential downsides that must be carefully weighed against its benefits. In this chapter, we will delve into the possible pitfalls of the Carnivore Diet, from nutrient deficiencies and long-term sustainability to ethical and environmental concerns. Additionally, we will consider the criticisms levelled by the medical and nutrition communities, offering a comprehensive perspective that empowers you to make informed decisions.

Nutrient Deficiencies: A Critical Concern

One of the primary criticisms of the Carnivore Diet is the potential for nutrient deficiencies. By excluding all plant-based foods, followers of this diet may miss out on essential vitamins, minerals, and fibre that are abundant in fruits, vegetables, grains, and legumes.

Vitamin C and Scurvy

Vitamin C, a crucial antioxidant, is predominantly found in fruits and vegetables. Its absence in a strictly meat-based diet raises concerns about the risk of scurvy, a disease caused by vitamin C deficiency. While some proponents argue that the body's requirement for vitamin C decreases on a low-carb diet due to reduced oxidative stress, this claim remains contentious and lacks substantial scientific backing.

Fibre and Digestive Health

Dietary fibre, found exclusively in plant foods, plays a vital role in maintaining digestive health. Fibre aids in bowel regularity, supports beneficial gut bacteria, and helps prevent conditions such as diverticulitis and colorectal cancer. The Carnivore Diet's lack of fibre can lead to digestive issues such as constipation and may negatively impact long-term gut health.

Vitamins and Minerals

Certain vitamins and minerals, such as magnesium, potassium, and vitamin K2, are more readily available in plant foods. While animal products provide many essential nutrients, the absence of a diverse diet can lead to imbalances and deficiencies. For instance, magnesium, crucial for muscle function and cardiovascular health, is abundant in leafy greens and nuts but less so in meat.

Sustainability and Long-Term Health Impacts

Another significant concern is the long-term sustainability and health impacts of the Carnivore Diet. While short-term benefits are often reported, the effects of adhering to this diet over many years are still largely unknown.

Heart Health and Saturated Fats

The high intake of saturated fats on the Carnivore Diet has raised alarms among health professionals. Historically, saturated fats have been linked to increased cholesterol levels and a higher risk of cardiovascular disease. Although recent research suggests that the relationship between saturated fats and heart disease is more complex, the long-term impact of consuming large quantities of animal fats remains a subject of debate.

Bone Health and Calcium

There is also concern about the diet's impact on bone health. High protein intake can increase calcium excretion in urine, potentially affecting bone density. While proponents argue that the body adapts to higher protein levels without adverse effects on bones, the lack of calcium-rich plant foods in the Carnivore Diet could pose risks, especially for individuals already at risk for osteoporosis.

Kidney Function

The high protein content of the Carnivore Diet may strain the kidneys, particularly in individuals with pre-existing kidney conditions. Proteins generate waste products that the kidneys must filter out, and excessive protein intake can exacerbate kidney damage. It is crucial for individuals with kidney issues to consult healthcare professionals before adopting such a diet.

Ethical and Environmental Concerns

Beyond individual health, the Carnivore Diet raises ethical and environmental questions that resonate with broader societal and cultural values.

Animal Welfare

The Carnivore Diet's reliance on animal products inevitably leads to concerns about animal welfare. Industrial farming practices, which often involve cramped and inhumane conditions, are a significant ethical issue. Advocates for humane treatment of animals argue that the demand for meat can perpetuate these unethical practices.

Environmental Impact

Livestock farming is a major contributor to greenhouse gas emissions, deforestation, and water usage. The environmental footprint of a meat-heavy diet is generally larger than that of a plant-based diet. While some proponents advocate for sourcing meat from regenerative agriculture practices, which aim to reduce environmental impact, these practices are not yet widespread. The sustainability of a global shift towards the Carnivore Diet is thus a contentious issue.

Sustainability of Resources

Feeding a growing global population with a predominantly meat-based diet could exacerbate resource depletion. Meat production requires more land, water, and energy compared to plant-based foods. The question of whether such a diet can be sustained on a large scale without further environmental degradation remains unanswered.

Criticisms from the Medical and Nutrition Communities

The Carnivore Diet faces significant criticism from many medical and nutrition experts, who argue that it is overly restrictive and may pose health risks.

Lack of Dietary Diversity

A common critique is that the Carnivore Diet lacks the diversity that is a cornerstone of many dietary guidelines. Diverse diets are believed to provide a wider range of nutrients and health benefits. The exclusion of entire food groups raises concerns about the diet's ability to meet all nutritional needs comprehensively.

Potential for Disordered Eating

The extreme restriction of food groups in the Carnivore Diet can lead to disordered eating patterns. This diet's rigid nature might foster an unhealthy relationship with food and create challenges in social and familial contexts. The potential psychological impact of such restrictive eating is an important consideration.

Unproven Long-Term Benefits

Critics highlight the lack of long-term studies on the Carnivore Diet. While short-term benefits are often reported, the long-term health impacts remain uncertain. Many health experts caution against adopting such a restrictive diet without more robust scientific evidence supporting its safety and efficacy over extended periods.

Addressing Criticisms and Mitigating Risks

Despite these criticisms, many proponents of the Carnivore Diet believe that its benefits outweigh the potential risks. Here are some strategies to address common concerns and mitigate risks:

Incorporating Nutrient-Rich Foods

Focus on a variety of nutrient-dense animal products, including organ meats, which are rich in vitamins and minerals. This can help address potential deficiencies. For instance, liver is a powerhouse of essential nutrients, including vitamin A, iron, and B vitamins.

Supplementation

Consider supplements to fill potential nutrient gaps, such as vitamin C, magnesium, and omega-3 fatty acids. Consult with a healthcare provider to determine appropriate supplementation. This proactive approach can help ensure that nutritional needs are met while following the Carnivore Diet.

Regular Monitoring

Regular health check-ups and monitoring of key health markers (such as cholesterol levels, kidney function, and bone density) can help detect and address potential issues early. Staying informed about your health status allows for timely adjustments to the diet if necessary.

Ethical Sourcing

Choose meat from sustainable and ethical sources. Supporting regenerative agriculture and small-scale, humane farming practices can reduce the environmental impact and ethical concerns associated with the diet. This conscientious approach aligns dietary choices with broader values of sustainability and animal welfare.

Flexibility and Balance

While the Carnivore Diet is inherently restrictive, some individuals might benefit from incorporating occasional plant foods or adopting a cyclical approach, where periods of strict carnivory are alternated with more inclusive eating patterns. This flexibility can help maintain a balanced relationship with food and reduce the risk of nutrient deficiencies.

Conclusion: A Balanced Perspective

The Carnivore Diet, like any dietary approach, comes with potential risks and criticisms that need to be carefully considered. While it offers numerous health benefits and has transformed the lives of many, it is not without its challenges and controversies. Understanding these potential risks and addressing them proactively is crucial for anyone considering or currently following the Carnivore Diet.

In the next chapter, we will explore how to get started on the Carnivore Diet, offering practical advice on transitioning, meal planning, and overcoming common challenges. Join us as we delve into the steps needed to embark on this unique dietary journey successfully.

FIVE | Getting Started on the Carnivore Diet

Embarking on a Carnivorous Journey: A Practical Guide

Transitioning to the Carnivore Diet is a transformative journey that requires careful planning and commitment. As with any significant lifestyle change, preparation and knowledge are key to ensuring a smooth and successful transition. This chapter provides practical advice on making the switch, including essential foods, meal planning, overcoming common challenges, and tips for monitoring your health and progress.

Essential Foods: Building Your Carnivore Pantry

The foundation of the Carnivore Diet lies in its simplicity and focus on animal-based foods. Stocking your pantry with the right essentials is the first step in your carnivorous journey. Here are some of the core foods to include:

Meat

Beef: A staple of the Carnivore Diet, beef is rich in protein and healthy fats. Cuts like ribeye, sirloin, and ground beef are versatile and nutrient dense.

Pork: *Pork provides variety and includes cuts such as pork chops, bacon, and sausages. Ensure your sausages are free from fillers and additives.*

Lamb: *Lamb is an excellent source of essential nutrients and offers a distinct flavour. Cuts like lamb chops and leg of lamb are popular choices.*

Poultry: *Chicken and turkey are leaner options that still offer substantial protein. Incorporate thighs, breasts, and wings into your meals.*

Seafood

Fish: *Fatty fishlike salmon, mackerel, and sardines are rich in omega-3 fatty acids, which support heart and brain health.*

Shellfish: *Shrimp, scallops, and oysters add variety and are excellent sources of protein and minerals.*

Organ Meats

Liver: *Often referred to as nature's multivitamin, liver is packed with essential vitamins and minerals. Beef liver is particularly nutrient-dense.*

Kidneys, Heart, and Other Offal: *These organ meats provide a range of nutrients and can be included to diversify your diet.*

Dairy and Eggs

Eggs: *Eggs are versatile and nutrient-rich, offering protein, healthy fats, and essential vitamins. They can be incorporated into various meals throughout the day.*

Cheese: *While some Carnivore Diet followers choose to avoid dairy, cheese can add flavour and variety. Opt for high-quality, full-fat cheeses.*

Fats

Butter and Ghee: *These fats are ideal for cooking and adding richness to your meals.*

Tallow and Lard: *Rendered animal fats are great for frying and can enhance the flavour of your dishes.*

Meal Planning: Crafting a Carnivore Menu

Effective meal planning is essential for maintaining variety and ensuring nutritional adequacy on the Carnivore Diet. Here's how to create a balanced and enjoyable carnivorous menu:

Breakfast

- **Scrambled Eggs with Bacon:** A classic breakfast that's easy to prepare and satisfying
- **Omelette with Cheese and Ham:** Customize your omelette with different cheeses and meats for variety.

- **Steak and Eggs:** A hearty option that provides ample protein and fats to start your day.

Lunch

- **Grilled Chicken Thighs:** Simple and flavourful, grilled chicken thighs can be seasoned with salt and pepper.
- **Beef Patties with Cheese:** Home-made beef patties topped with cheese offer a quick and nutritious lunch.
- **Shrimp Sautéed in Butter:** A lighter option that's rich in protein and healthy fats.

Dinner

- **Ribeye Steak with Garlic Butter:** A succulent ribeye steak topped with garlic-infused butter makes for a satisfying dinner.
- **Roast Lamb with Rosemary:** Roast lamb seasoned with rosemary and garlic is both flavourful and nutritious.
- **Pork Chops with a Side of Bone Broth:** Pork chops paired with nourishing bone broth provide a comforting meal.

Snacks and Supplements

- **Hard-Boiled Eggs:** Convenient and portable, hard-boiled eggs make for a perfect snack.
- **Cheese Cubes:** Pre-cut cheese cubes offer a quick and tasty snack option.
- **Bone Broth:** Sipping on bone broth can help maintain hydration and provide additional nutrients.

Overcoming Common Challenges

Transitioning to the Carnivore Diet can present several challenges, especially in the initial stages. Here are some common obstacles and strategies to overcome them:

Carb Withdrawal and Keto Flu:

As your body adapts to the absence of carbohydrates, you may experience symptoms commonly referred to as the "keto flu." These can include fatigue, headaches, and irritability.

Hydration and Electrolytes:

Stay Hydrated: *Drink plenty of water throughout the day to stay hydrated.*

Electrolyte Balance: *Ensure adequate intake of electrolytes such as sodium, potassium, and magnesium. Consider using electrolyte supplements if needed.*

Cravings for Carbohydrates:

Cravings for carbohydrates can be intense in the early stages of the Carnivore Diet. Here's how to manage them:

Eat Enough Fat: *Ensure your meals are rich in healthy fats, which can help reduce cravings.*

Stay Satisfied: *Eat until you feel full, focusing on nutrient-dense animal products.*

Find Alternatives: *When cravings strike, reach for carnivore-friendly* *snacks like bacon or cheese.*

Social Situations and Eating Out

Navigating social situations and dining out can be challenging. Here are some tips to stay on track:

Plan Ahead: *Review restaurant menus in advance and choose places that offer meat-based options.*

Communicate Your Needs: *Don't hesitate to ask for modifications to dishes, such as removing sauces or substituting sides with extra meat.*

Bring Your Own Food: *For gatherings and events, consider bringing your own carnivore-friendly dishes to ensure you have something to eat.*

Monitoring Your Health and Progress

Regularly monitoring your health and progress is crucial to ensure the Carnivore Diet is working for you and to make any necessary adjustments. Here are some tips:

Track Your Biometrics

Blood Tests: *Regular blood tests can help monitor cholesterol levels, kidney function, and other key health markers.*

Body Measurements: *Track changes in weight, body fat percentage, and* *muscle mass to gauge your physical progress.*

Blood Sugar Levels: *If you have diabetes or insulin resistance, regularly monitor your blood sugar levels to ensure they remain stable.*

Listen to Your Body

Energy Levels: *Pay attention to your energy levels throughout the day. Adjust your intake of protein and fats based on how you feel.*

Mental Clarity: *Note any changes in mental clarity and cognitive function, as these can be indicators of how well the diet is working for you.*

Digestive Health: *Monitor your digestive health and make adjustments if you experience any issues such as constipation or bloating.*

Adjusting Your Diet

Variety: *Ensure you're consuming a variety of meats and organ meats to obtain a broad spectrum of nutrients.*

Supplements: *If necessary, incorporate supplements to address any nutrient gaps, such as vitamin D, omega-3 fatty acids, and magnesium.*

Hydration: *Maintain proper hydration and electrolyte balance, especially if you're active or live in a hot climate.*

Conclusion: Your Path to Carnivorous Success

Transitioning to the Carnivore Diet is a significant lifestyle change that requires dedication and careful planning. By stocking your pantry with essential foods, crafting balanced and enjoyable meals, overcoming common challenges, and regularly monitoring your health, you can set yourself up for success on this unique dietary journey.

In the next chapter, we will explore a variety of meal plans and recipes to keep your carnivorous diet both nutritious and exciting. Join us as we delve into creative ways to prepare and enjoy meat-based meals, ensuring that your diet remains sustainable and satisfying.

SIX | Meal Plans and Recipes

The Art of Carnivorous Cuisine

Embarking on the Carnivore Diet doesn't mean sacrificing variety and flavour. On the contrary, this dietary approach can be incredibly diverse and delicious when you explore the myriad ways to prepare and enjoy meat-based meals. A successful Carnivore Diet relies on variety and proper preparation, ensuring you receive all the necessary nutrients while keeping your palate satisfied. This chapter offers sample meal plans, recipes, and cooking tips to keep your diet enjoyable and nutritious. From steak and burgers to organ meats and bone broth, you'll find plenty of delicious options to explore.

Sample Meal Plans: Structuring Your Carnivorous Day

Creating a meal plan is essential for maintaining variety and ensuring nutritional adequacy. Here's a sample weekly meal plan to inspire your carnivorous journey:

Monday:

- **Breakfast:** Scrambled eggs with bacon and a side of smoked salmon.
- **Lunch:** Grilled chicken thighs with a dollop of butter.
- **Dinner:** Ribeye steak cooked in garlic butter, served with a side of bone

marrow.

Tuesday:

- **Breakfast:** Omelette with cheese and diced ham.
- **Lunch:** Beef liver sautéed in ghee.
- **Dinner:** Pork chops with a side of shrimp sautéed in butter.

Wednesday:

- **Breakfast:** Hard-boiled eggs and a slice of aged cheddar cheese.
- **Lunch:** Pan-seared salmon with lemon and dill.
- **Dinner:** Slow-cooked lamb shanks with a rich bone broth gravy.

Thursday:

- **Breakfast:** Poached eggs with a side of sausage links.
- **Lunch:** Ground beef patties topped with melted cheese.
- **Dinner:** Grilled duck breast with a side of chicken liver pâté.

Friday:

- *Br***eakfast:** Carnivore waffles (made with pork rinds and eggs) topped with butter.
- **Lunch:** Tuna steaks seared in ghee.
- **Dinner:** Roast leg of lamb with a side of beef heart slices.

Saturday:

- **Breakfast:** Scrambled eggs with cream cheese and smoked bacon.
- **Lunch:** Grilled ribeye steak with a side of bone broth.
- **Dinner:** BBQ pork ribs cooked until tender.

Sunday:

- **Breakfast:** Cheese and egg muffins.
- **Lunch:** Roast chicken with crispy skin.
- **Dinner:** Seared scallops with a side of lamb kidneys.

Recipes: Carnivorous Delights

Here are some easy and delicious recipes to inspire your Carnivore Diet meals.

Beef Liver Pâté

Ingredients:

- 1/2-pound (225g) beef liver, cleaned and trimmed
- 1/4 cup (60ml) heavy cream or butter (for a richer texture)
- 1/2 teaspoon salt
- 1/4 teaspoon black pepper
- *Optional: a splash of apple cider vinegar for added flavour (if allowed)*

Instructions:

1. **Prepare the Liver:** Rinse the liver under cold water and pat dry. Trim any connective tissue.
2. **Cook the Liver:** Heat a skillet over medium heat and add some butter or animal fat. Cook the liver for about 3-4 minutes on each side until browned and cooked through.
3. **Blend the Pâté:** Transfer the cooked liver to a blender or food processor. Add the heavy cream or additional butter, salt, and pepper. Blend until smooth and creamy. Adjust seasoning to taste.

4. **Serve:** Serve the pâté with your grilled steak. You can also add a garnish of chopped chives or parsley for extra flavour if you prefer.

Garlic Butter

Ingredients:

- 2 tablespoons butter
- 2 cloves garlic, minced

Instructions:

1. In a small saucepan, melt the butter over medium heat and add the minced garlic. Cook until fragrant, about 1 minute.

Seared Bone Marrow

Ingredients:

- 2 to 4 beef marrow bones, cut lengthwise or crosswise
- Salt and pepper to taste

Instructions:

1. **Preheat the Oven:** Preheat your oven to 450°F (230°C).
2. **Prepare the Bones:** Place the marrow bones on a baking sheet, cut side up. Season with salt and pepper.
3. **Roast the Bones:** Roast in the oven for about 15-20 minutes until the marrow is soft and bubbling.

4. **Serve:** Serve the roasted marrow with your grilled steak. You can scoop out the marrow and spread it on the steak or eat it alongside.

Bone Broth

Ingredients:

- 2 to 3 lbs (900 to 1360g) beef bones (marrow bones, knuckles, etc.,)
- 1 tablespoon apple cider vinegar
- Water to cover the bones
- Salt to taste

Instructions:

1. Place the beef bones in a large pot or slow cooker.
2. Add the apple cider vinegar and enough water to cover the bones.
3. Bring to a boil, then reduce to a simmer. Skim off any foam that rises to the top.
4. Simmer for 12-24 hours, adding water as needed to keep the bones submerged.
5. Strain the broth, season with salt, and store in the refrigerator or freezer.

Egg Muffins

Ingredients:

- 8 large eggs
- 1/2 cup (120ml) heavy cream
- 1 cup (115g) shredded cheese (cheddar, mozzarella, or your favourite)

- Salt and pepper to taste
- Butter or animal fat for greasing the muffin tin
- **Optional:** Cooked Bacon, Ham or Sausage bits.

Instructions:

1. Preheat your oven to 375°F (190°C).
2. Grease a 12-cup muffin tin generously with butter or animal fat to prevent sticking.
3. In a large mixing bowl, crack the eggs and whisk them together with the heavy cream until well combined.
4. Season with salt and pepper.
5. Add the shredded cheese and optional meat
6. Pour the mixture into the prepared muffin tin, filling each cup about 3/4 full. The mixture should yield around 12 muffins.
7. Place the muffin tin in the preheated oven and bake for 20-25 minutes, or until the egg muffins are set and slightly golden on top.
8. Allow the muffins to cool for a few minutes before removing them from the tin. Serve warm.

Storage Tips:

Refrigerate: Store any leftovers in an airtight container in the refrigerator for up to 4-5 days. Reheat in the microwave or oven before serving.

Freeze: These muffins can also be frozen. Wrap each muffin individually in plastic wrap and store them in a freezer-safe bag for up to 2 months. Reheat in the microwave or oven before serving.

These carnivore-friendly egg muffins are a delicious and convenient option for breakfast or a quick snack, packed with protein and flavour.

Here are some tips to enhance your carnivorous cooking experience:

Use High-Quality Ingredients

- **Grass-Fed and Pasture-Raised:** Whenever possible, choose grass-fed and pasture-raised meats. These options are often higher in nutrients and healthier fats.
- **Fresh Seafood:** Opt for wild-caught seafood, which tends to have a better nutrient profile compared to farmed varieties.

Master Basic Techniques

- **Grilling:** Grilling is an excellent way to cook steaks, chops, and seafood, adding a smoky flavour and crisp texture.
- **Slow Cooking**: Slow cooking is perfect for tougher cuts of meat like brisket, pork shoulder, and lamb shanks, breaking down the fibres to create tender, flavourful dishes.
- **Pan-Seared Perfection:** For a quick and delicious meal, pan-searing cuts like steaks, liver, and fish fillets can create a beautiful crust while keeping the inside tender.

Experiment with Seasoning

- **Salt and Pepper:** High-quality sea salt and freshly ground black pepper are essential for seasoning your meats.
- **Herbs and Spices:** While some carnivores choose to avoid seasoning, incorporating herbs like rosemary, thyme, and garlic can enhance flavours without compromising the diet's principles.

Incorporate Organ Meats

- **Nutrient Powerhouses:** Organ meats like liver, kidneys, and heart are incredibly nutrient-dense. Start by incorporating small amounts into your meals and gradually increase as you become accustomed to the flavours.
- **Blending:** If the taste of organ meats is too strong, consider blending them with ground beef for meatballs or burgers.

Hydration and Electrolytes

- **Stay Hydrated:** Drinking plenty of water is crucial, especially when following a high-protein diet.
- **Electrolyte Balance:** Maintaining electrolyte balance is essential. Consider drinking bone broth or using electrolyte supplements to prevent dehydration and electrolyte imbalances.

Conclusion: Culinary Creativity on the Carnivore Diet

The Carnivore Diet, while seemingly restrictive, offers a world of culinary creativity and flavour. By planning your meals, experimenting with different cuts of meat, and mastering essential cooking techniques, you can enjoy a diverse and satisfying diet. The sample meal plans and recipes provided in this chapter are just the beginning. Embrace your inner chef and discover the endless possibilities of carnivorous cuisine.

In the next chapter, we will explore how to integrate exercise with the Carnivore Diet, optimizing your physical performance and recovery. Join us as we delve into the relationship between diet and fitness, offering insights and strategies for achieving your health and fitness goals on the Carnivore

Diet.

SEVEN | Exercise and the Carnivore Diet

Unleashing Physical Potential: Exercise and the Carnivore Diet

Physical activity is an essential component of a healthy lifestyle, providing numerous benefits that range from improved cardiovascular health to enhanced mental well-being. Integrating exercise into the Carnivore Diet can amplify these benefits, creating a synergy that promotes optimal health and peak performance. This chapter explores how to incorporate various types of workouts into your Carnivore Diet routine, supported by real-life success stories that illustrate the transformative power of this dietary approach.

Understanding the Synergy: Carnivore Diet and Physical Activity

The Carnivore Diet, rich in high-quality proteins and fats, provides the essential nutrients required for muscle repair, growth, and overall physical performance. Here's how this dietary approach supports different aspects of physical fitness:

Enhanced Muscle Protein Synthesis

Proteins are the building blocks of muscles. The Carnivore Diet, being protein-centric, ensures a steady supply of amino acids necessary for muscle protein synthesis. This is crucial for muscle growth, repair, and recovery, particularly after intense workouts.

Efficient Energy Utilization

Fats, the primary energy source in the Carnivore Diet, provide a sustained and efficient fuel supply. Unlike carbohydrates, which can cause energy spikes and crashes, fats offer a stable energy level, crucial for endurance activities and prolonged physical exertion.

Reduced Inflammation

Animal-based foods, particularly those rich in omega-3 fatty acids (like fatty fish), have anti-inflammatory properties. Reducing inflammation can enhance recovery, reduce muscle soreness, and improve overall performance.

Types of Workouts and Recommendations

To fully harness the benefits of the Carnivore Diet, it's important to incorporate a variety of workouts into your routine. Here are recommendations for different types of physical activities:

Strength Training

Strength training involves exercises that improve muscular strength and endurance. Examples include weightlifting, bodyweight exercises, and resistance band workouts.

Carnivore Diet Benefits:

Muscle Growth: High protein intake supports muscle hypertrophy and strength gains.

Recovery: Nutrient-dense animal foods aid in faster recovery and reduced muscle soreness.

Recommended Exercises:

Weightlifting: Incorporate compound movements such as squats, deadlifts, and bench presses. These exercises engage multiple muscle groups and promote overall strength.

Bodyweight Exercises: Push-ups, pull-ups, and planks are effective bodyweight exercises that can be done anywhere.

Cardiovascular Exercise

Cardiovascular (cardio) exercise improves heart and lung function. Examples include running, cycling, swimming, and rowing.

Carnivore Diet Benefits:

Sustained Energy: Fats provide a steady energy supply, enhancing endurance during prolonged cardio sessions.

Fat Utilization: The body becomes efficient at burning fat for fuel, beneficial for long-distance activities.

Recommended Exercises:

Running: Incorporate interval training and long-distance runs to build endurance and speed.

Cycling: Both outdoor cycling and stationary biking are excellent for cardiovascular health.

Swimming: A full-body workout that improves cardiovascular fitness and builds muscle.

High-Intensity Interval Training (HIIT)

HIIT involves short bursts of intense exercise followed by brief rest periods. It's effective for burning fat, improving cardiovascular health, and enhancing metabolic function.

Carnivore Diet Benefits:

Metabolic Boost: The diet supports high metabolic rates, crucial for burning calories during and after HIIT sessions.

Quick Recovery: Efficient nutrient absorption aids in quick recovery between intense intervals.

Recommended Exercises:

Sprint Intervals: Alternate between sprinting and walking or jogging.

Circuit Training: Combine exercises like burpees, jump squats, and kettlebell swings in quick succession.

Flexibility and Mobility Training

Flexibility and mobility exercises improve the range of motion, prevent injuries, and support overall physical health. Examples include yoga, stretching routines, and dynamic movements.

Carnivore Diet Benefits:

Joint Health: Nutrients like collagen, found in bone broth and connective tissues, support joint health.

Recovery: Reduced inflammation promotes quicker recovery and reduced stiffness.

Recommended Exercises:

Yoga: Incorporate yoga sessions to improve flexibility, balance, and mental clarity.

Dynamic Stretching: Perform dynamic stretches before workouts to enhance mobility and prevent injuries.

Real-Life Success Stories

Hearing from those who have successfully integrated the Carnivore Diet with their fitness routines can be both inspiring and informative. Here are some real-life success stories that illustrate the potential of this dietary approach.

John's Transformation: From Fatigue to Fitness

John, a 35-year-old software engineer, struggled with chronic fatigue and weight gain. Despite trying various diets and exercise regimens, he couldn't achieve his desired results. Upon discovering the Carnivore Diet, John decided to give it a try, combining it with a structured weightlifting program.

Within months, John experienced a significant transformation. He lost 40 pounds, gained muscle mass, and noticed a dramatic improvement in his energy levels. His strength increased, and he was able to lift heavier weights than ever before. John credits the Carnivore Diet for providing the necessary nutrients to fuel his workouts and recover effectively.

Sarah's Story: Overcoming Autoimmune Challenges

Sarah, a 28-year-old nurse, battled with autoimmune issues that left her feeling weak and in constant pain. Exercise seemed like an impossible task. After researching various dietary approaches, she decided to try the Carnivore Diet, hoping it would alleviate her symptoms and allow her to regain her strength.

Sarah started with gentle exercises like walking and yoga, gradually incorporating more strength training as her energy improved. The Carnivore Diet helped reduce her inflammation, and she began to feel stronger and more capable. Over time, Sarah was able to participate in high-intensity workouts and even completed a half-marathon, something she never thought possible.

Mark's Marathon Success

Mark, a 40-year-old avid runner, had always relied on carbohydrates to fuel his long-distance runs. However, frequent energy crashes and digestive issues led him to explore the Carnivore Diet. Sceptical at first, he decided to transition slowly, incorporating more animal-based foods and reducing his carb intake.

To his surprise, Mark found that his endurance improved, and he no longer experienced the energy dips that plagued his runs. He completed several marathons, achieving personal best times. The steady energy from fats and the anti-inflammatory benefits of the diet played a crucial role in his success.

Integrating Exercise into Your Carnivore Routine

To maximize the benefits of exercise while following the Carnivore Diet, consider these tips:

Prioritize Protein and Fat Intake

Ensure you're consuming enough protein to support muscle repair and growth. Include a variety of meats, seafood, and organ meats to cover all your nutritional bases. Healthy fats are equally important for sustained energy.

Stay Hydrated

Proper hydration is essential, especially when engaging in physical activity. Drink plenty of water throughout the day and consider electrolyte supplements to maintain balance.

Listen to Your Body

Pay attention to how your body responds to different exercises. Adjust your routine based on your energy levels and recovery needs. It's essential to find a balance that allows you to push your limits while ensuring adequate recovery.

Warm-Up and Cool Down

Incorporate warm-up exercises before your workouts to prepare your muscles and prevent injuries. Likewise, cooling down and stretching post-workout can aid in recovery and reduce muscle stiffness.

Consistency is Key

Regular exercise, combined with the Carnivore Diet, can lead to significant improvements in health and fitness. Consistency is crucial, so find activities you enjoy and make them a regular part of your routine.

Conclusion: Empowering Your Physical Potential

The synergy between the Carnivore Diet and physical exercise can unlock new levels of health and performance. By providing your body with the essential nutrients it needs and engaging in a variety of workouts, you can achieve your fitness goals and enhance your overall well-being. The real-life success stories shared in this chapter demonstrate the transformative power of this approach, offering inspiration and practical insights.

In the next chapter, we will explore how the Carnivore Diet can be adapted for specific populations, including athletes, older adults, and individuals with chronic illnesses. Join us as we delve into tailored strategies that ensure everyone can benefit from this unique dietary approach.

EIGHT | Carnivore Diet for Specific Populations

Tailoring the Carnivore Diet to Meet Unique Needs

While the Carnivore Diet offers a robust framework for health and wellness, it's important to recognize that different populations have unique nutritional needs and challenges. Athletes, women, older adults, and individuals with chronic illnesses may require specific adaptations to ensure the diet supports their health goals effectively. This chapter provides tailored advice to help these groups thrive on the Carnivore Diet.

Athletes: Fuelling Performance and Recovery

Athletes require optimal nutrition to support rigorous training schedules, enhance performance, and expedite recovery. The Carnivore Diet can be particularly beneficial due to its high protein content and nutrient density.

Protein for Muscle Repair and Growth

Protein is crucial for muscle repair and growth, especially for athletes engaging in strength training and endurance sports. The Carnivore Diet, rich in high-quality animal proteins, provides the necessary amino acids to support these processes. Athletes should focus on incorporating a variety of protein sources, including beef, chicken, fish, and organ meats.

Fat for Sustained Energy

Athletes often have high energy demands, and fats provide a dense and stable source of energy. Incorporating fatty cuts of meat, such as ribeye steak, salmon, and pork belly, ensures a steady fuel supply for prolonged physical activity.

Electrolyte Balance

Intense training can lead to significant electrolyte loss through sweat. To maintain electrolyte balance, athletes should consider consuming bone broth and using electrolyte supplements to replenish sodium, potassium, and magnesium levels.

Pre- and Post-Workout Nutrition

For optimal performance, athletes may benefit from specific pre- and post-workout nutrition strategies. Consuming a protein-rich meal or snack before training can provide the necessary fuel, while a post-workout meal can aid in recovery. Options include:

- **Pre-Workout:** A small serving of beef jerky or boiled eggs.

· **Post-Workout:** Grilled chicken breast with a side of bone broth.

Women: Addressing Hormonal and Nutritional Needs

Women have distinct nutritional needs, particularly related to hormonal health, pregnancy, and menopause. The Carnivore Diet can be adapted to support these needs effectively.

Hormonal Balance

Animal products provide essential fats and cholesterol, which are precursors for hormone production. Incorporating nutrient-dense foods like liver, eggs, and fatty fish can support hormonal balance and overall reproductive health.

Menopause

Menopausal women may experience changes in metabolism, bone density, and cardiovascular health. The Carnivore Diet's high protein content can help maintain muscle mass, while calcium-rich foods like sardines and bone-in cuts of meat support bone health. Additionally, the anti-inflammatory properties of omega-3-rich fish can benefit heart health.

Older Adults: Maintaining Vitality and Health

As we age, maintaining muscle mass, bone density, and overall vitality becomes increasingly important. The Carnivore Diet can be tailored to support these aspects of health in older adults.

Protein for Muscle Maintenance

Sarcopenia, or age-related muscle loss, is a common concern among older adults. Consuming sufficient protein is crucial for preserving muscle mass and strength. Including a variety of protein sources, such as beef, pork, and poultry, can help meet these needs.

Bone Health

Older adults are at higher risk of osteoporosis and fractures. Nutrients like calcium, vitamin D, and vitamin K2 are essential for bone health. Incorporating bone broth, sardines with bones, and liver can provide these nutrients.

Digestive Health

Digestive efficiency can decline with age, making it important to choose easily digestible foods. Ground meats, slow-cooked dishes, and broths are gentle on the digestive system and can help older adults absorb nutrients more effectively.

Individuals with Chronic Illnesses: Managing Health Conditions

The Carnivore Diet may offer therapeutic benefits for individuals with chronic illnesses, but it's essential to adapt the diet to address specific health concerns.

Autoimmune Diseases

For individuals with autoimmune diseases, reducing inflammation is a key goal. The Carnivore Diet's elimination of potentially inflammatory plant foods can help manage symptoms. Including anti-inflammatory foods like fatty fish and organ meats can provide additional benefits. However, it's important to work with a healthcare provider to monitor the condition and adjust the diet as needed.

Diabetes

The Carnivore Diet's low carbohydrate content can help stabilize blood sugar levels and improve insulin sensitivity, making it beneficial for individuals with diabetes. Monitoring blood sugar levels regularly and working with a healthcare provider to adjust medication and dietary intake is crucial. Focusing on fatty cuts of meat and organ meats can provide sustained energy without spiking blood sugar.

Heart Disease

For those with heart disease, prioritizing omega-3-rich foods like salmon and mackerel is important for their anti-inflammatory and heart-protective properties. Additionally, choosing leaner cuts of meat and incorporating moderate amounts of high-quality fats can help manage cholesterol levels and support cardiovascular health.

Customizing the Carnivore Diet: Practical Tips

To ensure the Carnivore Diet meets the unique needs of various populations, consider these practical tips:

Variety and Nutrient Density

Diversity within animal-based foods is key to obtaining a wide range of nutrients. Rotate different types of meat, seafood, and organ meats to cover all nutritional bases. For example, include beef liver for vitamin A, salmon for omega-3s, and eggs for choline.

Supplements

In some cases, supplements may be necessary to fill nutritional gaps. Common supplements for those on the Carnivore Diet include vitamin D, magnesium, and omega-3 fatty acids. Always consult with a healthcare provider before starting any supplementation.

Monitoring and Adjusting

Regular health check-ups and monitoring specific biomarkers, such as blood sugar levels, cholesterol, and kidney function, can help ensure the diet is supporting overall health. Adjustments may be needed based on individual health status and goals.

Listening to Your Body

Pay attention to how your body responds to the diet. Energy levels, digestive health, and overall well-being are important indicators of how well the diet is working for you. Make adjustments as needed to optimize your health and performance.

Personalization for Athletes

Athletes might need to tweak their macronutrient ratios, ensuring they get enough fat for sustained energy and protein for muscle repair. Incorporating organ meats can also help meet the increased micronutrient demands of intense training.

Women's Health Considerations

Women should focus on balancing hormone-supportive nutrients like healthy fats and cholesterol. Those who are pregnant or breastfeeding need to ensure they are getting enough calories and micronutrients to support both their own health and that of their baby.

Adaptations for Older Adults

Older adults might benefit from softer, easier-to-digest cuts of meat and the inclusion of broths and slow-cooked dishes that are gentle on the digestive system. Ensuring adequate hydration and monitoring for signs of dehydration is also important.

Managing Chronic Illnesses

Individuals with chronic illnesses should work closely with healthcare providers to tailor the Carnivore Diet to their specific needs. Regular monitoring and adjustments can help manage symptoms and support overall health.

Conclusion: Tailoring the Carnivore Diet for Optimal Health

The Carnivore Diet can be a powerful tool for enhancing health across different populations, but it requires thoughtful customization to meet unique nutritional needs and challenges. By focusing on variety, nutrient density, and regular monitoring, athletes, women, older adults, and individuals with chronic illnesses can thrive on this diet.

In the next chapter, we will explore the social and psychological aspects of the Carnivore Diet, providing strategies to navigate social situations, manage cravings, and maintain a positive relationship with food. Join us as we delve into the holistic aspects of adopting and sustaining the Carnivore Diet.

NINE | Social and Psychological Aspects

Navigating the Carnivore Diet in Social Landscapes

Adopting the Carnivore Diet can be a transformative journey for many, yet maintaining this dietary lifestyle in social contexts can present unique challenges. From dining out and attending social gatherings to managing cravings and coping with the psychological impacts of such a drastic dietary change, this chapter provides strategies to help you navigate these aspects with confidence and ease. Building a supportive community will also be emphasized, underscoring the importance of shared experiences and collective encouragement.

Dining Out: Strategies for Success

Dining out can be one of the most challenging aspects of maintaining a Carnivore Diet. However, with a bit of preparation and savvy decision-making, you can enjoy meals out without compromising your dietary principles.

Research and Plan Ahead

Before heading out to a restaurant, take some time to review the menu online. Many restaurants post their menus, allowing you to identify carnivore-friendly options in advance. Look for steakhouses, BBQ joints, and seafood restaurants, which typically offer a variety of meat-based dishes.

Communicate Your Needs

Don't hesitate to communicate your dietary preferences to the restaurant staff. Politely requesting modifications, such as removing sauces or substituting vegetable sides with extra meat, can help ensure your meal aligns with the Carnivore Diet. Most restaurants are willing to accommodate special requests, especially when explained clearly and courteously.

Simple Choices

Opt for simple, straightforward dishes that are less likely to include hidden ingredients. Grilled steaks, burgers without the bun, roasted chicken, and seafood platters are often safe bets. Avoid dishes with complex sauces or breading, which may contain non-carnivore ingredients.

Sample Scenario: A Night Out at a Restaurant

Imagine you're at an Italian restaurant with friends. While pasta dominates the menu, you notice a grilled ribeye steak with a side of vegetables. Politely ask the waiter if you can replace the vegetables with an extra serving of steak or a side of buttered shrimp. By making this request, you enjoy a satisfying, carnivore-compliant meal without drawing attention to your dietary restrictions.

Dealing with Cravings: Staying Strong

Cravings for non-carnivore foods, especially in the early stages of the diet, can be challenging. However, with the right strategies, you can manage and overcome these cravings.

Identify Triggers

Understanding what triggers your cravings is the first step in managing them. Common triggers include stress, boredom, social cues, and specific environments. By identifying these triggers, you can develop strategies to avoid or cope with them.

Satiate with Fat

Ensuring that you consume enough fat can help curb cravings. Fat is highly satiating and can prevent the hunger pangs that lead to cravings. Incorporate fatty cuts of meat, such as ribeye and pork belly, into your meals, and don't shy away from adding butter or ghee.

Carnivore-Friendly Snacks

Keep carnivore-friendly snacks on hand to combat cravings. Hard-boiled eggs, beef jerky, pork rinds, and cheese cubes can provide quick relief when cravings strike. Having these snacks readily available can prevent you from reaching for non-compliant foods.

Sample Scenario: Handling Late-Night Cravings

Suppose you're watching a movie late at night, and a sudden craving for popcorn hits. Instead of giving in, reach for a handful of beef jerky or a few slices of cheese. These snacks not only align with your diet but also provide the satisfaction of a tasty treat.

Psychological Aspects: Embracing the Change

The psychological impacts of adopting a restrictive diet like the Carnivore Diet can be significant. It's essential to address these aspects to maintain a healthy relationship with food and ensure long-term success.

Mindset Shift

Adopting the Carnivore Diet often requires a significant mindset shift. Embrace the idea that you're making a positive change for your health and well-being. Focus on the benefits you're experiencing, such as improved energy levels, mental clarity, and physical health, to reinforce your commitment to the diet.

Coping with Social Pressure

Social pressure can be a major obstacle, especially when friends and family don't understand or support your dietary choices. Prepare yourself for questions and comments by educating yourself about the diet and having thoughtful responses ready. Sharing your personal success and the benefits you've experienced can help others understand your decision.

Finding Joy in Simplicity

One of the keys to thriving on the Carnivore Diet is finding joy in the simplicity of your meals. Appreciate the flavours, textures, and satiation that high-quality animal products provide. By focusing on the positives, you can maintain a positive outlook and reduce the psychological burden of dietary restrictions.

Sample Scenario: Dealing with Family Gatherings

Imagine attending a family barbecue where the spread includes a variety of non-carnivore foods. Rather than feeling deprived, focus on the delicious options available to you, such as grilled steaks and chicken wings. Bring a carnivore-friendly dish to share, showcasing that your dietary choices are both enjoyable and sustainable.

Building a Supportive Community

Having a supportive community can make a significant difference in your journey on the Carnivore Diet. Whether it's online forums, local meetups, or social media groups, connecting with others who share your dietary approach provides encouragement, shared experiences, and practical advice.

Online Communities

Join online forums and social media groups dedicated to the Carnivore Diet. These platforms offer a wealth of information, from recipes and success stories to troubleshooting tips and moral support. Participating in these communities can help you feel connected and supported.

Local Meetups

Seek out or organize local meetups with other carnivores. These gatherings provide an opportunity to share experiences, exchange tips, and enjoy carnivore-friendly meals together. Building in-person connections can enhance your sense of community and commitment.

Support from Friends and Family

Educate your friends and family about your dietary choices and the reasons behind them. While they may not fully understand or embrace the Carnivore Diet, their awareness can foster a more supportive environment. Encourage open communication and express your appreciation for their support.

Sample Scenario: Joining an Online Community

Suppose you're feeling isolated in your Carnivore Diet journey. Joining an online community like a Facebook group dedicated to carnivorous eating can provide instant connection and support. Engage in discussions, share your progress, and learn from others' experiences to stay motivated and inspired.

Conclusion: Thriving Socially and Psychologically on the Carnivore Diet

Maintaining a Carnivore Diet in social situations and managing the psychological aspects of dietary change can be challenging, but it's entirely possible with the right strategies. By planning ahead, managing cravings, shifting your mindset, and building a supportive community, you can navigate these challenges and thrive on the Carnivore Diet.

In the next chapter, we will explore the future of the Carnivore Diet, considering advancements in nutritional science, cultural shifts, and the potential role of this diet in broader health and wellness trends. Join us as we look ahead to the evolving landscape of carnivorous eating.

TEN | The Future of the Carnivore Diet

Looking Ahead: The Evolution and Promise of the Carnivore Diet

As the Carnivore Diet continues to gain attention and followers, its future is shaped by ongoing research, emerging dietary guidelines, and its portrayal in popular culture. This chapter explores these dimensions, highlighting the potential for new insights and developments, as well as the challenges and opportunities that lie ahead.

Ongoing Research: Unveiling the Science

The Carnivore Diet, though supported by numerous anecdotal success stories, requires rigorous scientific validation to fully understand its benefits and risks. Current and future research will play a crucial role in shaping the perception and acceptance of this diet within the broader nutritional science community.

Metabolic Health and Weight Loss

One of the primary areas of interest is the diet's impact on metabolic health and weight loss. Preliminary studies suggest that low-carbohydrate, high-protein diets can be effective for weight management and improving insulin sensitivity. Ongoing research aims to elucidate the mechanisms by which the Carnivore Diet may contribute to these outcomes, focusing on hormonal regulation, fat metabolism, and appetite control.

Autoimmune and Chronic Diseases

The potential of the Carnivore Diet to manage autoimmune and chronic diseases is another promising avenue of research. Studies are investigating how an all-meat diet affects inflammation, gut health, and immune function. By examining the diet's impact on specific conditions such as rheumatoid arthritis, type 2 diabetes, and irritable bowel syndrome, researchers hope to provide evidence-based guidelines for its therapeutic use.

Nutrient Absorption and Bioavailability

Understanding nutrient absorption and bioavailability in the context of the Carnivore Diet is essential for assessing its long-term viability. Research is exploring how the absence of plant-based foods affects the absorption of vitamins and minerals, particularly those commonly associated with plants, such as vitamin C and magnesium. These studies aim to determine whether animal-based foods can sufficiently meet all nutritional requirements.

Potential Dietary Guidelines: Bridging Tradition and Modern Science

As scientific understanding of the Carnivore Diet evolves, so too might dietary guidelines that integrate its principles with broader nutritional recommendations. Potential guidelines could emphasize the following aspects:

Variety within Animal-Based Foods

Encouraging a diverse intake of animal-based foods, including muscle meats, organ meats, seafood, and eggs, can help ensure a comprehensive nutrient profile. Guidelines might also highlight the importance of sourcing high-quality, pasture-raised, and sustainably harvested products.

Supplementation Strategies

Given the potential for nutrient gaps, future guidelines might recommend strategic supplementation for certain vitamins and minerals. For example, vitamin D, magnesium, and omega-3 fatty acids could be highlighted as key supplements for individuals following the Carnivore Diet.

Periodic Health Monitoring

Regular health monitoring, including blood tests and physical assessments, could become a standard recommendation for those on the Carnivore Diet. This approach would help identify and address any emerging deficiencies or health concerns early on.

Dietary Flexibility

Acknowledging that strict adherence to the Carnivore Diet may not be suitable for everyone, guidelines could promote a more flexible approach. This might include periods of strict carnivory interspersed with the inclusion of select plant-based foods to enhance dietary balance and variety.

Popular Culture: Shaping Perception and Acceptance

The portrayal of the Carnivore Diet in popular culture significantly influences public perception and acceptance. As media coverage, social media influencers, and celebrities continue to spotlight this diet, its visibility and appeal grow.

Celebrity Endorsements

High-profile endorsements from celebrities and athletes have played a pivotal role in popularizing the Carnivore Diet. Public figures sharing their success stories and health transformations can inspire a broader audience to explore this dietary approach.

Documentaries and Media Coverage

Documentaries and media coverage that delve into the Carnivore Diet's principles, benefits, and controversies contribute to a more informed public dialogue. Balanced and well-researched portrayals can help dispel myths and provide a nuanced understanding of the diet's potential.

Social Media Influence

Social media platforms offer a space for individuals to share their Carnivore Diet experiences, recipes, and tips. These online communities foster a sense of belonging and support, encouraging more people to try and sustain the diet. However, it's important to critically evaluate the information shared on these platforms and seek evidence-based guidance.

Future Challenges: Navigating Obstacles

While the Carnivore Diet holds promise, several challenges must be addressed to ensure its credibility and sustainability.

Nutritional Adequacy

Ensuring nutritional adequacy remains a significant challenge. Critics argue that the exclusion of plant-based foods can lead to deficiencies in essential nutrients. Future research and guidelines must provide clear strategies to mitigate these risks, whether through dietary diversity within animal-based foods or appropriate supplementation.

Long-Term Health Effects

The long-term health effects of the Carnivore Diet are not yet fully understood. As more people adopt this dietary approach, longitudinal studies are needed to monitor health outcomes over extended periods. This data will be crucial for determining the diet's safety and efficacy.

Environmental and Ethical Considerations

The environmental impact of a meat-centric diet is a contentious issue. Sustainable farming practices and ethical sourcing are critical to addressing these concerns. Advocates of the Carnivore Diet must engage in discussions about reducing the environmental footprint and promoting animal welfare.

Healthcare and Professional Acceptance

Gaining acceptance within the healthcare and professional nutrition communities is another hurdle. Many healthcare providers remain sceptical of the Carnivore Diet due to the lack of comprehensive research and its deviation from established dietary guidelines. Bridging this gap requires robust scientific evidence and open dialogue between practitioners and proponents of the diet.

Future Opportunities: Expanding Horizons

Despite these challenges, the future of the Carnivore Diet is ripe with opportunities for growth and innovation.

Integrative Approaches

Integrating the Carnivore Diet with other dietary frameworks could offer a balanced approach to nutrition. For example, combining periods of carnivory with ketogenic or paleo principles might provide a more sustainable and nutrient-rich dietary pattern.

Personalized Nutrition

Advancements in personalized nutrition, driven by genetic and microbiome research, could tailor the Carnivore Diet to individual needs. Understanding how genetic variations and gut microbiota influence nutrient absorption and metabolism can help customize the diet for optimal health outcomes.

Education and Advocacy

Educational initiatives and advocacy efforts can promote a deeper understanding of the Carnivore Diet. By providing accurate information, resources, and support, advocates can empower individuals to make informed dietary choices.

Technological Innovations

Technological innovations, such as lab-grown meat and advancements in sustainable farming practices, have the potential to address environmental and ethical concerns. These developments could make high-quality, ethically produced animal products more accessible and environmentally friendly.

Conclusion: The Road Ahead

The Carnivore Diet stands at the intersection of tradition and innovation, offering a unique approach to health and nutrition. As research progresses and our understanding deepens, this diet has the potential to evolve and adapt, meeting the diverse needs of modern society.

While challenges remain, the opportunities for growth and improvement are vast. By embracing scientific inquiry, ethical considerations, and personalized approaches, the Carnivore Diet can continue to inspire and transform lives.

In the next chapter, we will provide practical tips for sustaining the Carnivore Diet long-term, ensuring that you have the tools and strategies needed for lasting success. Join us as we explore how to navigate this dietary journey with confidence and resilience.

BONUS | Sustaining the Carnivore Diet

Practical Tips for Long-Term Success

Embracing Longevity: Sustaining the Carnivore Diet

Adopting the Carnivore Diet can be a profound and life-changing experience, offering numerous health benefits and a simplified approach to nutrition. However, sustaining this diet for the long term requires strategic planning, resilience, and adaptability. This bonus chapter provides practical tips for maintaining the Carnivore Diet over time, ensuring that you can continue to thrive while embracing this unique dietary lifestyle.

Building a Sustainable Carnivore Routine

Creating a sustainable routine is essential for long-term success on the Carnivore Diet. This involves developing habits that make it easy to stick to the diet while meeting your nutritional needs and enjoying your meals.

Stock Your Pantry and Freezer

A well-stocked pantry and freezer are crucial for maintaining the Carnivore Diet. Ensure you have a variety of meats, seafood, and organ meats on hand to provide diversity and prevent dietary monotony.

Pantry Essentials:

- **Canned Meats:** Keep canned meats such as tuna, salmon, and sardines for quick and convenient meals.
- **Beef Jerky and Pork Rinds:** These are great for snacking and can be used as quick meal components.
- **Bone Broth:** Store bone broth for its nutritional benefits and as a base for soups and stews.

Freezer Essentials:

- **Bulk Purchases:** Buy meats in bulk and freeze them in portions for easy access.
- **Variety of Cuts:** Include different cuts of meat such as steaks, roasts, ground meat, and organ meats.
- **Seafood:** Keep a selection of frozen fish and shellfish to add variety and essential nutrients.

Meal Planning and Preparation

Effective meal planning and preparation can simplify your daily routine and ensure you always have carnivore-friendly meals ready.

Weekly Meal Prep:

- **Batch Cooking:** Prepare large batches of meat, such as roasting a whole chicken or slow cooking a beef roast, and portion them for the week.
- **Pre-Cut Portions:** Pre-cut and marinate meat portions for quick cooking during the week.

Daily Planning:

- **Breakfast:** Plan simple and quick options like scrambled eggs with bacon or a cheese and egg omelette.
- **Lunch:** Opt for easy-to-reheat meals such as leftover steak or grilled chicken.
- **Dinner:** Include a variety of protein sources, like lamb chops one night and salmon fillets the next.

Navigating Social Situations

Maintaining the Carnivore Diet in social settings can be challenging, but with the right strategies, you can stay on track while enjoying social interactions.

- **Dining Out:** Choose the Right Restaurants: Opt for steakhouses, BBQ joints, and seafood restaurants that offer meat-centric menus.
- **Customize Your Order:** Don't hesitate to ask for modifications, such as removing sauces or substituting sides with extra meat.
- **Social Gatherings:** Bring Your Own Dish: Bring a carnivore-friendly dish to share, ensuring you have something to eat and introducing others to your diet.
- **Communicate Your Needs:** Let the host know about your dietary preferences in advance to help accommodate your needs.

Travelling:

- **Pack Snacks:** Bring portable snacks like beef jerky, pork rinds, and cheese sticks to avoid non-carnivore options.
- **Research Ahead:** Look up restaurants and grocery stores at your destination to find carnivore-friendly options.

Dealing with Cravings and Dietary Boredom

Cravings and dietary boredom can be significant challenges when following a restrictive diet long-term. Here's how to manage and overcome them.

Addressing Cravings:

- **Satiate with Fat:** Ensure you're consuming enough fat to keep you full and satisfied, reducing the likelihood of cravings.
- **Carnivore Snacks:** Keep carnivore-friendly snacks on hand, such as hard-boiled eggs, bacon, and cheese.

Adding Variety:

- **Experiment with Cooking Methods:** Try different cooking methods like grilling, roasting, slow-cooking, and sous-vide to keep meals interesting.
- **Use Different Cuts and Types of Meat:** Rotate between different cuts of meat and include a variety of seafood and organ meats.
- **Seasoning and Sauces:** Use simple seasoning like salt, pepper, and herbs, and make carnivore-friendly sauces such as garlic butter or bone broth gravy.

Monitoring Your Health and Adjusting

Regularly monitoring your health and making necessary adjustments is crucial for long-term success on the Carnivore Diet.

Health Check-Ups:

- **Regular Blood Tests:** Monitor key health markers such as cholesterol levels, blood sugar, and kidney function.
- **Bone Density Scans:** Particularly important for older adults to ensure bone health.

Listening to Your Body:

- **Energy Levels:** Pay attention to your energy levels and adjust your protein and fat intake accordingly.
- **Digestive Health:** Monitor your digestive health and make adjustments if you experience issues like constipation or bloating.

Making Adjustments:

- **Supplementation:** Consider supplements if needed to address any deficiencies. Common supplements include vitamin D, magnesium, and omega-3 fatty acids.
- **Dietary Flexibility:** Be open to incorporating occasional plant foods if necessary to meet your nutritional needs while maintaining the core principles of the Carnivore Diet.

Building a Supportive Community

Having a supportive community can make a significant difference in sustaining the Carnivore Diet long-term. Here are ways to build and engage with a supportive network.

Online Communities:

Forums and Social Media Groups: Join online forums and social media groups dedicated to the Carnivore Diet. Engage in discussions, share experiences, and learn from others.

Local Support:

- **Meetups and Events:** Attend local meetups and events with fellow carnivores to share experiences and support each other.
- **Family and Friends:** Educate your family and friends about your dietary choices and seek their support and understanding.

Staying Informed and Motivated

Staying informed about new research and developments can help you stay motivated and confident in your dietary choices.

Continuous Learning:

- **Books and Articles:** Read books and articles about the Carnivore Diet to deepen your understanding and stay updated on the latest research.
- **Podcasts and Webinars:** Listen to podcasts and attend webinars featuring

experts and enthusiasts in the Carnivore community.

Setting Goals and Tracking Progress:

- **Set Realistic Goals:** Set achievable health and fitness goals to keep yourself motivated.
- **Track Your Progress:** Use a journal or app to track your dietary adherence, physical activity, and health improvements.

Conclusion: Thriving on the Carnivore Diet

Sustaining the Carnivore Diet for the long term is a journey that requires dedication, flexibility, and continuous learning. By building a sustainable routine, navigating social situations, managing cravings, monitoring your health, and engaging with a supportive community, you can thrive on this diet and enjoy its numerous benefits.

Remember that every individual's journey is unique, and it's important to listen to your body and make adjustments as needed. Embrace the simplicity and nourishment of the Carnivore Diet while staying open to new insights and developments.

As you continue on this path, you'll discover the full potential of the Carnivore Diet to enhance your health and well-being. Stay curious, stay informed, and most importantly, stay committed to your journey towards optimal health.

CONCLUSION

Embracing the Carnivore Journey: Reflections and Future
Pathways

As we conclude this comprehensive exploration of the Carnivore Diet, it is essential to reflect on the insights we've gathered and the transformative potential this dietary approach offers. From understanding its historical roots to navigating the complexities of modern nutrition science, we have delved into the many facets of the Carnivore Diet. Our journey has spanned the scientific underpinnings, the health benefits, the challenges, and the practical strategies needed for long-term success. This conclusion will synthesize these insights, reinforce the key takeaways, and inspire you to apply this knowledge in your pursuit of health and well-being.

A Return to Simplicity

At its core, the Carnivore Diet is a return to dietary simplicity. In a world where food choices are often overwhelming and confusing, this diet strips away the complexities, focusing on nutrient-dense, animal-based foods. This simplicity can be both liberating and empowering, offering a clear path to nutrition that our ancestors likely followed.

The historical context provided in Chapter 1 reminded us that early human diets were predominantly meat-based, laying the foundation for our evolution and survival. Traditional societies, such as the Inuit and Maasai, have thrived on meat-centric diets, showcasing the viability and health benefits of such an approach. This ancestral wisdom provides a compelling argument for revisiting and embracing a diet that aligns with our evolutionary heritage.

The Science of Nourishment

Chapters 2 and 3 delved into the science behind the Carnivore Diet, highlighting how this dietary approach impacts our metabolism, hormonal balance, and overall health. The emphasis on high-quality proteins and healthy fats supports muscle growth, brain function, and metabolic health. The state of ketosis, induced by carbohydrate restriction, offers a stable and efficient energy source, enhancing mental clarity and reducing inflammation.

Scientific research continues to explore the potential of the Carnivore Diet to manage chronic conditions, such as autoimmune diseases and diabetes. While more studies are needed to fully understand its long-term effects, the existing evidence and numerous testimonials underscore its therapeutic potential. By focusing on nutrient-dense foods, the Carnivore Diet provides essential vitamins and minerals in bioavailable forms, supporting overall health and vitality.

Health Benefits and Real-Life Transformations

The health benefits of the Carnivore Diet, as discussed in Chapter 3, are profound and varied. Weight loss improved mental clarity, and relief from chronic ailments are among the most commonly reported benefits. Real-life success stories, like those of John, Sarah, and Mark, illustrate the transformative power of this diet. These individuals have not only improved their physical health but also experienced enhanced energy levels, mental well-being, and quality of life.

John's journey from fatigue to fitness, Sarah's triumph over autoimmune challenges, and Mark's marathon successes serve as powerful testaments to the potential of the Carnivore Diet. Their stories inspire and motivate, demonstrating that with commitment and the right strategies, anyone can achieve remarkable health transformations.

Navigating Challenges and Criticisms

No diet is without its critics, and the Carnivore Diet is no exception. Chapter 4 addressed the potential risks and criticisms, including nutrient deficiencies, long-term sustainability, and ethical and environmental concerns. Acknowledging these challenges is crucial for making informed decisions and approaching the diet with a balanced perspective.

Ensuring nutritional adequacy through variety, supplementation, and regular health monitoring can mitigate many of the concerns associated with the Carnivore Diet. Ethical sourcing and sustainable farming practices address the environmental and animal welfare issues, promoting a more conscientious approach to meat consumption.

Practical Strategies for Success

Chapters 5 through 7 provided practical advice for getting started on the Carnivore Diet, meal planning, and integrating exercise. Building a sustainable routine, navigating social situations, and managing cravings are key to long-term adherence and success. Effective meal planning and preparation ensure dietary variety and satisfaction, while strategic exercise integration enhances physical performance and recovery.

The importance of building a supportive community, as highlighted in Chapter 9, cannot be overstated. Engaging with like-minded individuals, whether through online forums or local meetups, provides encouragement, shared experiences, and valuable insights. This sense of belonging and support can make a significant difference in sustaining the Carnivore Diet.

Adapting for Specific Populations

The adaptability of the Carnivore Diet for specific populations, such as athletes, women, older adults, and individuals with chronic illnesses, was explored in Chapter 8. Tailoring the diet to meet unique needs ensures that everyone can benefit from its principles. Athletes, for example, can optimize their performance and recovery by focusing on nutrient-dense, high-protein foods, while older adults can support muscle maintenance and bone health through careful food choices and supplementation.

Future Pathways and Opportunities

Looking ahead, the future of the Carnivore Diet is filled with opportunities for growth and innovation. Ongoing research will continue to shed light on its benefits and risks, guiding the development of more nuanced dietary guidelines. Integrative approaches, personalized nutrition, and technological advancements in sustainable farming and lab-grown meat hold promise for addressing current challenges and enhancing the diet's viability.

The portrayal of the Carnivore Diet in popular culture, through documentaries, media coverage, and celebrity endorsements, will shape public perception and acceptance. Balanced and well-researched portrayals can help dispel myths and promote a more informed dialogue about the diet's potential.

Empowering Your Journey

As you embark on or continue your Carnivore Diet journey, remember that it is a deeply personal and evolving experience. Listen to your body, stay informed, and remain open to adjustments and new insights. The Carnivore Diet is not a one-size-fits-all solution, but a flexible framework that can be adapted to meet your unique needs and goals.

Embrace the simplicity, nourishment, and transformative potential of this diet. Celebrate your successes, learn from challenges, and connect with others who share your path. The knowledge and strategies provided in this book are tools to empower you, guiding you towards optimal health and well-being.

Final Reflections

In closing, the Carnivore Diet represents a return to dietary simplicity and a profound reconnection with our ancestral roots. It challenges conventional wisdom and offers a unique approach to health that is both empowering and liberating. By understanding its principles, benefits, and challenges, and by applying practical strategies for long-term success, you can harness the full potential of the Carnivore Diet.

As you move forward, may you find joy in the simplicity of your meals, strength in the nourishment they provide, and inspiration in the transformative power of this dietary journey. Remember, the pursuit of health is a lifelong endeavour, and the Carnivore Diet is but one path among many. Stay curious, stay committed, and most importantly, stay true to yourself and your health goals.

Thank you for joining me on this exploration of the Carnivore Diet. May your journey be filled with health, vitality, and a deeper understanding of the profound connection between what we eat and how we live.

REFERENCES

Cordain, L., Eaton, S. B., Sebastian, A., Mann, N., Lindeberg, S., Watkins, B. A., O'Keefe, J. H., & Brand-Miller, J. (2005). Origins and evolution of the Western diet: health implications for the 21st century. The American Journal of Clinical Nutrition, 81(2), 341-354. doi:10.1093/ajcn.81.2.341

Baker, S. (2018). The Carnivore Diet. Victory Belt Publishing.

Peterson, M. (2019). The Lion Diet: How Eating Meat Only Saved My Life. Retrieved from Mikhaila Peterson Blog

Cordain, L. (2011). The Paleo Answer: 7 Days to Lose Weight, Feel Great, Stay Young. John Wiley & Sons.

Stefansson, V. (1946). Not By Bread Alone. Macmillan.

Eaton, S. B., & Konner, M. (1985). Paleolithic nutrition. A consideration of its nature and current implications. New England Journal of Medicine, 312(5), 283-289. doi:10.1056/NEJM198501313120505

Volek, J. S., & Phinney, S. D. (2011). The Art and Science of Low Carbohydrate Living. Beyond Obesity LLC.

Paoli, A., Rubini, A., Volek, J. S., & Grimaldi, K. A. (2013). Beyond weight loss: a review of the therapeutic uses of very-low-carbohydrate (ketogenic) diets. European Journal of Clinical Nutrition, 67(8), 789-796. doi:10.1038/ejcn.2013.116

Saladino, P. (2020). The Carnivore Code: Unlocking the Secrets to Optimal Health by Returning to Our Ancestral Diet. Houghton Mifflin Harcourt.

Hallberg, S. J., Gershuni, V. M., Hazbun, T. L., & Athinarayanan, S. J. (2019). Reversing Type 2 Diabetes: A Narrative Review of the Evidence. Nutrients, 11(4), 766. doi:10.3390/nu11040766

Goldberg, E. L., & Dixit, V. D. (2015). Ketogenic diet: Celebrated but not yet fully understood. Diabetes, 64(3), 719-721. doi:10.2337/db14-1606

Mikhaila Peterson Blog. (2019). The Lion Diet: How Eating Meat Only Saved My Life. Retrieved from Mikhaila Peterson Blog

Katz, D. L., & Meller, S. (2014). Can we say what diet is best for health? Annual Review of Public Health, 35, 83-103. doi:10.1146/annurev-publhealth-032013-182351

Ioannidis, J. P. A. (2018). The challenge of reforming nutritional epidemiologic research. JAMA, 320(10), 969-970. doi:10.1001/jama.2018.11025

The Lancet. (2019). Food in the Anthropocene: the EAT–Lancet Commission on healthy diets from sustainable food systems. The Lancet, 393(10170), 447-492. doi:10.1016/S0140-6736(18)31788-4

Wolf, R. (2010). The Paleo Solution: The Original Human Diet. Victory Belt Publishing.

Taubes, G. (2007). Good Calories, Bad Calories: Fats, Carbs, and the Controversial Science of Diet and Health. Alfred A. Knopf.

Phinney, S. D., & Volek, J. S. (2012). The Art and Science of Low Carbohydrate Performance. Beyond Obesity LLC.

Kresser, C. (2013). Your Personal Paleo Code: The 3-Step Plan to Lose Weight, Reverse Disease, and Stay Fit and Healthy for Life. Little, Brown Spark.

Shanahan, C. (2016). Deep Nutrition: Why Your Genes Need Traditional Food. Flatiron Books.

Wolf, R. (2019). Wired to Eat: Turn Off Cravings, Rewire Your Appetite for Weight Loss, and Determine the Foods That Work for You. Harmony.

Fitzgerald, M. (2018). 80/20 Running: Run Stronger and Race Faster By Training Slower. Penguin Random House.

Sisson, M., & Kearns, B. (2017). Primal Endurance: Escape chronic cardio and carbohydrate dependency and become a fat burning beast!. Bradventures LLC.

Kraemer, W. J., & Ratamess, N. A. (2004). Fundamentals of resistance training: progression and exercise prescription. Medicine and Science in Sports and Exercise, 36(4), 674-688. doi:10.1249/01.MSS.0000121945.36635.61

Laquale, K. M. (2016). Nutrition for Athletes. Current Sports Medicine Reports, 15(4), 252-257. doi:10.1249/JSR.0000000000000272

Tulchinsky, T. H. (2010). Micronutrient deficiency conditions: global health issues. Public Health Reviews, 32(1), 243-255.

Drewnowski, A., & Evans, W. J. (2001). Nutrition, physical activity, and quality of life in older adults: summary. Journals of Gerontology Series A: Biological Sciences and Medical Sciences, 56(Special Issue 2), 89-94. doi:10.1093/gerona/56.suppl_2.89

Adams, T. B., Moore, M. T., & Dye, J. (2007). The relationship between physical activity and mental health in a national sample of college females. Women & Health, 45(1), 69-85. doi:10.1300/J013v45n01_05

Herman, C. P., & Polivy, J. (2008). External cues in the control of food intake in humans: the sensory-normative distinction. Physiology & Behavior, 94(5), 722-728. doi:10.1016/j.physbeh.2008.04.014

Baumeister, R. F., & Leary, M. R. (1995). The need to belong: desire for interpersonal attachments as a fundamental human motivation. Psychological Bulletin, 117(3), 497-529. doi:10.1037/0033-2909.117.3.497

Ludwig, D. S., & Ebbeling, C. B. (2018). The Carbohydrate-Insulin Model of Obesity: Beyond "Calories In, Calories Out". JAMA Internal Medicine, 178(8), 1098-1103. doi:10.1001/jamainternmed.2018.2933

Arnett, D. K., Blumenthal, R. S., Albert, M. A., Buroker, A. B., Goldberger, Z. D., Hahn, E. J., Himmelfarb, C. D., Khera, A., Lloyd-Jones, D., McEvoy, J. W., Michos, E. D., Miedema, M. D., Muñoz, D., Smith, S. C., Virani, S. S., Williams, K. A., Yeboah, J., & Ziaeian, B. (2019). 2019 ACC/AHA Guideline on the Primary Prevention of Cardiovascular Disease: A Report of the American College of Cardiology/American Heart Association Task Force on Clinical Practice Guidelines. Journal of the American College of Cardiology, 74(10), e177-e232. doi:10.1016/j.jacc.2019.03.010

Willett, W. C., Sacks, F., Trichopoulou, A., Drescher, G., Ferro-Luzzi, A., Helsing, E., & Trichopoulos, D. (1995). Mediterranean diet pyramid: a cultural model for healthy eating. The American Journal of Clinical Nutrition, 61(6 Suppl), 1402S-1406S. doi:10.1093/ajcn/61.6.1402S

Saslow, L. R., Mason, A. E., Kim, S., Goldman, V., Ploutz-Snyder, R., Bayan-dorian, H., Daubenmier, J. J., Hecht, F. M., Moskowitz, J. T. (2017). An Online Intervention Comparing a Very Low-Carbohydrate Ketogenic Diet and Lifestyle Recommendations Versus a Plate Method Diet in Overweight Individuals with Type 2 Diabetes: A Randomized Controlled Trial. Journal of Medical Internet Research, 19(2), e36. doi:10.2196/jmir.5806

Urbain, P., Strom, L., Morawski, L., Bertz, H. (2016). Impact of a 6-month very-low-carbohydrate diet on metabolic health in individuals with type 2 diabetes. Diabetic Medicine, 33(5), 662-670. doi:10.1111/dme.12833

Volek, J. S., Noakes, T., & Phinney, S. D. (2015). The Real Meal Revolution: The Radical, Sustainable Approach to Healthy Eating. Little, Brown and Company.